THIS I BELIEVE

Frederick K. Slicker

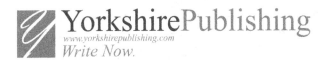

YorkshirePublishing
www.yorkshirepublishing.com
Write Now.

ISBN: 978-1-936750-96-2
Published by Yorkshire Publishing, LLC
9731 East 54th Street
Tulsa, OK 74146

This I Believe
4444 East 66th Street. Suite 201
Tulsa, OK 74136-4206

Cover Design: Luke Owens

Requests for consent may be made to Frederick K. Slicker, 4444 Est 66th Street, Suite 201, Tulsa, Oklahoma 74136-4206, telephone 918-496-9020, fax 918-496-9024, e-mail: fred@slickerlawfirm.com.

Index

Dedication

This I Believe is dedicated to my wife, Claudia, my daughter, Laura, my son, Kipp, and to their families in the hope that they too will come to believe in a very deep, real and personal way that Jesus is the Christ, their Lord and Savior, and that they too can trust Him with all they have and all they are. To God be the Glory!

Introduction

There is an old classic song that starts: "I believe that for every drop of rain that falls, a flower grows..." There is hope in believing, there is peace in believing and there is comfort in knowing what you believe. But what do I believe?

In the movie, *Bull Durham,* Kevin Costner played an aging minor league catcher, Crash Davis, brought down to a Single A league team to teach the meaning of baseball to the latest phenom, Luke Laloosh. Susan Sarandon plays Annie, the team's groupie who chooses one player each year with whom to be monogamous for the season to teach him the ways of the world. Annie selects Crash and Luke to try out for her affections. As Crash was leaving her home late one evening, Annie asks Crash, "What do you believe?" He answers in part: "I believe in a hanging curve and a long slow kiss at midnight." Everyone believes something, but few of us take the time to focus on what we believe, why we believe it or how those beliefs make a difference in our lives and in the lives of those around us.

"What do I believe?" **I have come to believe and to know with certainty that there is a loving God, that He made me for a purpose, that He loves me, even when I ignore or reject Him, and that He is waiting patiently for me to surrender who I am to Him, so that He can use me and bless others through me for His purposes.**

Like millions before me, my journey of faith began without my knowledge or consent at infant baptism on All Saints Eve, October 31, 1943, when I was 2 months old. This act of faith by my parents planted a seed within me and set me on a life long quest to find the heart of God.

The ministry of Jesus began after He was baptized and received the affirmation from His Father: "This is my beloved Son, in whom I am well pleased." At that moment, doves descended upon Jesus, all heaven rejoiced and the Holy Spirit was released for use by Jesus in His ministry. Immediately following His baptism, Jesus selected his first disciples: Fishermen, not high priests, not holy men and not Biblical scholars. These ordinary fishermen became extraordinary witnesses to the world and started a revolution that continues today. One day the entire world will bow down and worship Jesus, because they believe Jesus is the Son of the Living God, the Savior of the World.

In Part I, I state what I think I believe. In Part II, I test my preliminary statements of belief against what the eye witnesses in the Book of John did to test their beliefs. In Part III, I consider my preliminary beliefs against the statements of belief by some of the most famous and celebrated scholars, philosophers, theologians and creative thinkers throughout the history of mankind. I also consider the wisdom of Solomon in Ecclesiastes and statements of belief by famous and ordinary Americans from the *This I Believe Project.* In Part IV, I examine my preliminary beliefs against my experiences and my current battle with cancer. In Part V, I conclude with some thoughts about the River of Life which flows from

God's throne to provide all of God's blessings to man. The River symbolizes and summarizes what I believe.

In seeking God, my journey has taken many twists and turns, but incomprehensible grace, peace and joy beyond measure await me as I submit more to His will. I have concluded that God is in control of my life, that God made me for a purpose, and that God wants me to embrace Him with my whole heart. When I do, God showers me with blessings beyond belief, including God's peace, joy and grace.

THIS I BELIEVE.

TO GOD BE ALL THE GLORY!

Frederick K. Slicker
September 1, 2012

PART I:

WHAT I THINK I BELIEVE

What I Believe Generally

I believe:

My greatest honor has been to be the father of Laura and Kipp.
My greatest blessing is who Laura and Kipp have become.
My greatest joy has been being with Claudia, Laura and Kipp.
My greatest victory has been the joy of family.

I believe:

Rugged individualism must give way to shared community.
Individual freedoms come from shared sacrifices.
Free expression and exercise of religious beliefs are essential for a free society.
The rule of law survives only if equality, justice and fairness are achieved.

I believe:

Right is right, no matter who says differently.
Truth is truth, even if many deny it.
Justice and righteousness come from God.
God is good. God is great. All the time!

I believe:

Obstacles are opportunities to overcome.
Failure is temporary unless we fail to rise up.
Success is built upon character, truth and wisdom.
Truth and wisdom are gifts from God.

I believe:

Character matters.
Honesty matters.
Righteousness matters.
Integrity matters.
Simplicity matters.
Truth matters.

I believe in:

The power of words:
Words can hurt and heal.
Words can criticize and comfort.
Words can reject and embrace.
Words can condemn and bless.

I believe:

Passion trumps passivity.
Perseverance trumps passion.
Perspiration trumps inspiration.
Peace trumps possessions.

I believe:

Faithfulness to God brings joy and peace.
Pride is man's biggest fault.
Wisdom triumphs over power and prestige.
Fortune and fame are at best temporary.

I believe:

Science and faith are not inherently in conflict.
Science seeks to explain and duplicate the physical world.
Religion defines what is good and moral and sacred.
Faith believes in the unseen hand of God.
There is no Truth without God.

I believe:

Adversity provides opportunity.
Achievement requires overcoming long held beliefs.
Attitude gives meaning to purpose.
Affirmation produces loyalty.

I believe:

Life is a journey of individual moments.
Things happen for a reason.
Random events are not always random.
Defining moments can be divine moments.

I believe:

We cannot have mountains without valleys.
We cannot be bold without having been broken.
We cannot hear others unless we listen in silence.
We cannot feel compassion without sharing pain.

I believe:

Attitude is a matter of choice.
All choices have eternal consequences.
What we do is more important than what we say.
How we act is a reflection of what we believe.

I believe:

The rule of law is America's greatest gift to mankind.
The rule of law is necessary to restrain man's pride.
The rule of law works only if it protects fundamental
freedoms.
The rule of law requires respect for fundamental fairness.

I believe:

Midnight is always followed by the dawn.
Darkness always gives way to the Light.
Joy always comes to the humble.
Peace always comes from surrender.

I believe:

Pride pollutes the goodness of man.
Individual achievement leads to pride.
Humility is the key to surrender.
Surrender to God is the primary duty of man.

I believe in:

The mystery of miracles.
The existence of angels and demons.
The awe of signs and wonders.
The presence of God at all times in all places.

I believe:

Without trials, there can be no victories.
Without pain, there can be no gain.
Without listening, there is no understanding.
Without loss, there can be no love.

I believe:

Giving is a double blessing:
One to the recipient; the other to the donor.
Forgiveness is a double blessing:
One to the forgiven; the other to the one forgiving.

I believe:

Kindness is always rewarded in kind.
Service is the key to significant living.
Truth always finds a way of becoming known.
Wisdom follows experience and compassion.

I believe in:

Praising in public.
Encouraging in public.
Affirming in public.
Correcting in private.

I believe:

Taking issue with people produces conflict.
Taking issue with positions produces understanding.
Taking issue with policies leads to enlightenment.

I believe:

Wrong is wrong, no matter who disagrees.
Right is right, even if many people disagree.
There is no right way to do a wrong thing.
Doing wrong to achieve a right is always wrong.

I believe:

Human beings are spiritual beings.
Each person has a divine call and purpose.
Seeking purpose reveals divine meaning.
Finding meaning comes from accepting God's grace.

See *A Treasury of Truth and Wisdom* by Frederick K. Slicker, Yorkshire Publishing (2007) for other statements of general belief.

What I Believe Spiritually

I believe:

There is one true God, Creator of all:
King of kings, Lord of lords;
Abba Father, the Great I AM;
Perpetually present, always available.

I believe:

Before the stars were, God existed.
Before the void was, God filled it.
Before time began, God created it.
Before life, God imagined it.

I believe:

God is.
God is holy.
God comes.
God calls.

I believe:

God gives.
God cares.
God knows.
God loves me anyway.

I believe:

God invites.
God embraces.
God forgives.
God forgets.

I believe:

God lives in me.
God is with me.
God is for me.
God loves me.

I believe:

God is Spirit.
God is Light.
God is Love.
God is Life.

I believe:

God is holy.
God is sacred.
God is alive.
God is perpetually available.

I believe:

God is all knowing.
God is all powerful.
God is always present.
God is always available.

I believe:

God's Word calls me to believe.
God's Word calls me to obey.
God's Word calls me to surrender.
God's Word calls me to care.

I believe:

Jesus is the Word of God.
Jesus is the Son of God.
Jesus is the Messiah.
Jesus is my Lord and Savior.

I believe:

God is the Author of all life.
God is present with me at all times.
God created me for a purpose.
God cares for me personally.

I believe:

God gives me a choice.
God trusts me to believe.
God knows my deepest thoughts.
God loves me anyway.

I believe:

God is Light.
Light dispels the darkness.
Where Light is, darkness flees.
Light reveals the Truth.

I believe:

Grace cannot be bought.
Grace cannot be earned.
Grace cannot be stored up.
Grace is a gift from God.

I believe:

We were made to seek God.
We were made to worship God.
We were made to praise God.
We can trust God with our all.

I believe:

Peace is only possible when God is in it.
Joy only comes when we find God.
Forgiveness brings freedom.
The peace of God passes all understanding.

I believe:

God's love is present.
God's love is permanent.
God's love is personal.
God's love is perpetual.

I believe:

There are two world systems constantly colliding:
One consists of everything that is not God.
The other consists of everything that is of God.
Which world we choose to reside in dictates our destiny.

I believe:

There are demons and angels all around.
There are no accidents, coincidences or random events.
Everyone and everything is connected.
God is in control of it all.

I believe:

"It is not with swords loud clashing,
Nor roll of stirring drums,
But simple acts of kindness,
That the heavenly kingdom comes."

I believe:

Choice is God's gift to man.
Choice comes with consequences.
The quality of our choices determines the quality of our lives.
Choosing God always results in joy, peace and life.

I believe:

God gives power to the powerless.
God gives hope to the hopeless.
God gives healing to the sick.
God gives peace to the troubled.

I believe:

God gives love to the loveless.
God gives comfort to the disturbed.
God gives poise to the troubled.
God gives life to the dead.

I believe:

God gives wisdom to the humble.
God gives direction to the lost.
God gives purpose to the troubled.
God gives joy to all who believe in Him.

I believe in:

The wonder of words.
The joy of grace.
The power of prayer.
The blessings of belief.

I believe:

Confession is the key to forgiveness.
Forgiveness is the key to redemption.
Surrender is the prerequisite to freedom.
Wholeness and holiness come only from God.

I believe:

We are standing on holy ground.
We are in His presence at all times.
We are blessed beyond belief.
We are His, even if we ignore Him.

I believe:

In the end, what we believe defines our character.
In the end, what we do reflects who we are.
In the end, all things return to God.
In the end, God's peace prevails.

I believe in the Apostles' Creed:

> I believe in God the Father Almighty,
> maker of heaven and earth;
> And in Jesus Christ His Only Son our Lord;
> who was conceived by the Holy Spirit,
> born of the Virgin Mary,
> suffered under Pontius Pilate,
> was crucified, dead and buried;
> the third day He rose from the dead;
> He ascended into heaven,
> and sits at hand right hand of God the Father Almighty;
> from thence He shall come to judge the quick and
> the dead.
> I believe in the Holy Spirit,
> The holy catholic church,
> The communion of saints,
> The forgiveness of sins,
> The resurrection of the body,
> And the life everlasting.

I also believe these words from the Service of Resurrection contained in the *United Methodist Hymnal*:

> Dying, Christ destroyed death.
> Rising, Christ restored our life.
> Christ will come again in glory.
> As in baptism, I put on Christ,
> so in Christ may I be clothed with glory.
> Here and now, dear friends, we are God's children.
> What we shall be has not yet been revealed;
> but we know that when He appears,
> we shall be like Him,
> for we shall see Him as He is.
> Those who have this hope purify themselves
> as Christ is pure.

PART II:

BELIEVE: THE GOSPEL OF JOHN

Believe: The Gospel of John

The Gospel of John is all about *believing*. John uses the term *believed* eighteen times, *believes* thirteen times and *believe* forty-four times. More than any other book in the Bible, the Book of John asserts that *believing* is the key to living now and for eternity. The Gospel of John was written for a specific purpose:

"Jesus did many other miraculous signs in the presence of his disciples, which are not recorded in this book. But these are written that you may **believe that Jesus is the Christ, the Son of God, and that by believing you may have life in his name.**" John 20:30–31

Some People Believed, because Others Claimed Jesus Was the Christ.

John the Baptist said that Jesus is the "One and Only Son of God." John 1:18

John the Baptist said that Jesus is the "Lamb of God." John 1:29

Peter said that Jesus is the "Holy One of God." John 6:69

The Samaritan woman at the well called Him the "Messiah." John 4:25–26

The Samaritan crowds called Him the "Savior of the World."
John 4:42

John said that Jesus is the "Christ, the Son of God."
John 20:30

The crowds called Him "Teacher," "Rabbi," "Prophet" and
"Lord." John 8:4; John 1:38; John 7:40; and John 6:68

Some People Believed because of the Miracles Jesus Did.

Jesus performed seven specific miracles as described in the
Book of John:

Jesus turned water into wine. John 2:1–11

Jesus healed the royal official's son. John 4:46–54

Jesus healed the cripple at the Bethesda pool outside the city.
John 5:1–15

Jesus fed the multitudes. John 6:1–14

Jesus walked on water. John 6:16–21

Jesus gave sight to the blind man. John 9:1–4

Jesus raised Lazarus from the dead. John 11:1–44

John writes in closing that there were many other miracles that occurred that were not described, because the "whole world would not have room for the books that would be written if every one of them were written down." John 21:25

Some People Believed because of the Prophesies Jesus Made Which Later Occurred.

Jesus predicted the betrayal by Judas. John 13:19

Jesus predicted His own death. John 16:27

Jesus predicted His crucifixion. John 14:29

Jesus predicted His resurrection. John 11:25

Jesus predicted the coming of the Holy Spirit. John 16:8–9

Jesus predicted that Peter would deny Him three times. John 18:17, 25, 27

Jesus predicted that the disciples would scatter. John 16:30–31

Some People Believed because of Who Jesus Said He Is.

Jesus said that He is the "the bread of life." John 6:35

Jesus said that He is "the Way, the Truth and the Life." John 14:6

Jesus said that no one comes to the Father except through Jesus. John 14:7

Jesus said that He is the "light of the world." John 3:19–20

Jesus said that He is "the Resurrection and the Life." John 11:25

Jesus said that He is the "gate" to God and the "good shepherd." John 10:9–11

Jesus said that He is the "true vine." John 15:1

Jesus said that He is the "temple of God." John 16:11

Jesus said that He is the "living water." John 4:10

Jesus said that He is the "one whom God sent into the world." John 3:34

Jesus said that He and the "Father are One." John 10:30

Speaking to Nicodemus, Jesus said: "Just as Moses lifted up the snake in the desert, so the Son of Man must be lifted up, that everyone who *believes* in him may have eternal life. For God so loved the world that he gave his one and only Son, that whoever *believes* in him shall not perish but have eternal life." John 3:15–16

The Samaritans said to the woman at the well, "We no longer *believe* just because of what you said; now we have heard for ourselves, and we know that this man really is the Savior of the world." John 4:41–42

Speaking to the Jewish leaders, Jesus said: "I tell you the truth, whoever hears my word and *believes* him who sent me has eternal life and will not be condemned." John 5:24

To the crowds at Capernaum, Jesus declared: "I am the bread of life. He who comes to me will never go hungry, and he who *believes* in me will never be thirsty." John 6:33, 35

To the crowds at Capernaum, Jesus said: "For my Father's will is that everyone who looks to the Son and *believes* in him shall have eternal life, and I will raise him up at the last day." John 6:40

Teaching in the temple, Jesus said: "'Whoever *believes* in me, as the Scripture has said, streams of living water will flow from within him.' By this he meant the Spirit whom those who *believed* in him were later to receive." John 7:38–39

To the Jews who *believed*, Jesus said: "If you hold to my teachings, you are really my disciples. Then you will know the truth, and the truth will set you free." John 8:31

To the Jews who were stoning him, Jesus said: "Do not *believe* me unless I do what my Father does. But if I do it, even though you do not *believe* me, *believe* the miracles that you may know and understand that the Father is in me, and I in the Father." John 10:37–38

To the crowds, Jesus cried out, "When a man *believes* in me, he does not *believe* in me only, but in the one who sent me…I have come into the world as a light, so that no one who *believes* in me should stay in darkness." John 12:44, 46

Some People Believed, because They Experienced His Blessing Directly.

Jesus gave sight to the blind man. John 9:1–4

To the blind man he healed, Jesus said, "Do you *believe* in the Son of Man?" "Who is he, sir?" the man asked. "Tell me so that I may *believe* in him." Jesus said, "You have now seen him; in fact, he is the one speaking with you." Then the man said, "Lord, I *believe*," and he worshipped him. John 9:35–38

Jesus raised Lazarus from the dead. John 11:1–44

Jesus said to the disciples: "Peace be with you." Then he said to Thomas, "Put your finger here; see my hands. Reach out your hand and put it into my side. Stop doubting and *believe*." Thomas said to him, "My Lord and my God!" Then Jesus told him, "Because you have seen me, you have *believed*; blessed are those who have not seen and yet have *believed*." John 20:27–29

Jesus healed the royal official's son.

"Then [the royal official] realized that this was the exact time at which Jesus had said to him:

"Your son will live." So he and all his household *believed.*"
John 4:53

Some People Believed because of the Resurrection of Jesus.

"After he was raised from the dead, his disciples recalled what
he had said. Then they *believed* the Scripture and the words
that Jesus had spoken." John 2:22

Jesus said to Martha, "I am the resurrection and the life.
He who *believes* in me will live, even though he dies; and
whoever lives and *believes* in me will never die. Do you
believe this?" "Yes, Lord," she told him, "I *believe* that you
are the Christ, the Son of God, who was to come into the
world." John 11:25–27

"Finally, the other disciple [John] who had reached the tomb
first also went inside. He saw and *believed.*" John 20:8

"So the other disciple [John] told him [Thomas], 'We have
seen the Lord.' But he [Thomas] said to them, 'Unless I see
the nail marks in his hands and put my finger where the nails
were, and put my hand into his side, I will not *believe* it.'"
John 20:25

Jesus said to the disciples: "Peace be with you." Then he said
to Thomas, "Put your finger here; see my hands. Reach out
your hand and put it into my side. Stop doubting and *believe.*"
Thomas said to him, "My Lord and my God!" Then Jesus
told him, "Because you have seen me, you have *believed*;

blessed are those who have not seen and yet have *believed.*"
John 20:27–29

But Sadly Some People Never Believed at All.

Jesus said to his disciples: "The Spirit gives life; the flesh counts for nothing. The words I have spoken to you are spirit and they are life. Yet there are some of you who do not *believe.*" John 6:63–64

"For even his own brothers did not *believe* in him." John 7:5

To the Pharisees and teachers of the law, Jesus said: "I told you that you would die in your sins; if you do not *believe* that I am the one I claim to be, you will indeed die in your sins." John 8:24

To the Jews that did not believe, Jesus said: "Yet because I tell you the truth, you do not *believe* me! Can any of you prove me guilty of sin? If I am telling the truth, why don't you *believe* me?" John 8:45-46

The Pharisees and the chief priests said to the Sanhedrin: "If we let him go on like this, everyone will *believe* in him, and then the Romans will come and take away both our place and our nation." John 11:48

Jesus said to Phillip: "Don't you *believe* that I am in the Father, and that the Father is in me? The words I say to you are not just my own. Rather, it is the Father living in me who is doing his work. *Believe* me when I say that I am in the Father and the Father is in me, or at least *believe* on the evidence of the miracles themselves." John 14:10–11

"Yet at the same time many even among the Jewish leaders *believed* in him. But because of the Pharisees, they would not confess their faith for fear they would be put out of the synagogue. For they loved praise from men more than praise from God." John 12:42

Believe: The Core of John

The Book of John is all about **believing**. There are seventy-five specific references in John to **believing**.

John: Passage:

1:7   "He [John] came as a witness to testify concerning that light, so that through him all men might **believe**."

1:12   "Yet to all who received him, to those that **believed** in his name, he gave the right to become children of God."

1:50   Jesus said [to Nathanael]: "You **believe** because I told you I saw you under the fig tree."

2:22   "After he was raised from the dead, his disciples recalled what he had said. Then they **believed** the Scripture and the words that Jesus had spoken."

2:23   Now while he was in Jerusalem at the Passover Feast, many people saw the miraculous signs he was doing and **believed** in his name.

3:12   [Jesus said to Nicodemus]: "I have spoken to you of earthly things and you do not **believe**; how then will you **believe** if I speak of heavenly things?"

John: Passage:

3:15–16   [Speaking to Nicodemus, Jesus said]: "Just as
           Moses lifted up the snake in the desert, so the
           Son of Man must be lifted up, that everyone who
           believes in him may have eternal life. For God so
           loved the world that he gave his one and only Son,
           that whoever *believes* in him shall not perish but
           have eternal life."

3:18   [Speaking to Nicodemus, Jesus said]: "Whoever
           believes in him is not condemned, but whoever
           does not *believe* stands condemned already because
           he has not *believed* in the name of God's one and
           only Son."

3:36   [Speaking of Jesus to the crowds, John said]:
           "Whoever *believes* in the Son has eternal life, but
           whoever rejects the Son will not see life, for God's
           wrath remains on him."

4:21   Jesus declared [to the woman at the well]: "*Believe*
           me, woman, a time is coming when you will
           worship the Father neither on this mountain nor
           in Jerusalem."

4:39   "Many of the Samaritans from the town *believed* in
           him because of the woman's testimony."

4:41   "And because of his [Jesus'] words many more
           became *believers.*"

John: Passage:

4:42   They [the Samaritans] said to the woman, "We no longer *believe* just because of what you said; now we have heard for ourselves, and we know that this man really is the Savior of the world."

4:48   "Unless you people see miraculous signs and wonders," Jesus told [the royal official], "you will never *believe*."

4:53   "Then [the royal official] realized that this was the exact time at which Jesus had said to him, "Your son will live." So he and all his household *believed.*"

5:24   [Jesus to the Jewish leaders:] "I tell you the truth, whoever hears my word and *believes* him who sent me has eternal life and will not be condemned."

5:38   [Jesus to the Jewish leaders]: "You have never heard his voice nor seen his form, nor does his word dwell in you, for you do not *believe* the one he sent."

5:44   [Jesus to the Jewish leaders]: "How can you *believe* if you accept praise from one another, yet make no effort to obtain the praise that comes from the only God."

John: Passage:

5:46–47   [Jesus said to the Jewish leaders]: "If you **believed** Moses, you would **believe** me, for he wrote about me. But since you do not **believe** what he wrote, how are you going to **believe** what I say?"

6:29–30   [To his disciples:] Jesus answered, "The work of God is this: to **believe** in the one he has sent." So they asked him, "What miraculous sign then will you give that we may see it and **believe** you?"

6:35–36   Then Jesus declared [to the crowds at Capernaum]: "I am the bread of life. He who comes to me will never go hungry, and he who **believes** in me will never be thirsty. But as I told you, you have seen me and still you do not **believe**."

6:40   [Jesus said to the crowds at Capernaum]: "For my Father's will is that everyone who looks to the Son and **believes** in him shall have eternal life, and I will raise him up at the last day."

6:47   [Jesus said to the grumbling Jews]: "I tell you the truth, he who **believes** has everlasting life."

6:63–64   [Jesus said to his disciples]: "The Spirit gives life; the flesh counts for nothing. The words I have spoken to you are spirit and they are life. Yet there are some of you who do not **believe**."

John: Passage:

6:69   [Peter said]: "We *believe* and know that you are the
             Holy One of God."

7:5   "For even his own brothers did not *believe* in him."

7:38–39   [Teaching in the temple, Jesus said]: "Whoever
             believes in me, as the Scripture has said, streams
             of living water will flow from within him. By this
             he meant the Spirit whom those who *believed* in
             him were later to receive."

7:48   [The Pharisees said to the temple guards]: "Has
             any of the rulers of the Pharisees *believed* in him?
             No! But this mob that knows nothing of the law—
             there is a curse on them."

8:24   [To the Pharisees and teachers of the law, Jesus
             said]: "I told you that you would die in your sins;
             if you do not *believe* that I am the one I claim to be,
             you will indeed die in your sins."

8:31   "To the Jews who had *believed* him, Jesus said,
             'If you hold to my teachings, you are really my
             disciples. Then you will know the truth, and the
             truth will set you free.'"

John: Passage:

8:45–46 [To the Jews that did not *believe*, Jesus said]: "Yet because I tell you the truth, you do not *believe* me! Can any of you prove me guilty of sin? If I am telling the truth, why don't you *believe* me?"

9:18   "The Jews still did not *believe* that he had been blind and had received his sight until they sent for the man's parents."

9:35–38 "Jesus heard that they had thrown him [the blind man healed by Christ] out, and when he found him, he said, "Do you *believe* in the Son of Man?" "Who is he, sir?" the man asked. "Tell me so that I may *believe* in him." Jesus said, "You have now seen him; in fact, he is the one speaking with you." Then the man said, "Lord, I *believe*," and he worshipped him."

10:25–26 Jesus answered [the unbelieving Jews]: "I did tell you, but you do not *believe*. The miracles I do in my Father's name speak for me, but you do not *believe* because you are not my sheep."

10:37–38 [To the Jews who were stoning Jesus]: "Do not *believe* me unless I do what my Father does. But if I do it, even though you do not *believe* me, *believe* the miracles, that you may know and understand that the Father is in me, and I in the Father."

John: Passage:

10:41–42 "...and many people came to him [Jesus]: They said, 'Though John never performed a miraculous sign, all that John said about this man was true.' And in that place many *believed* in Jesus."

11:15   [To his disciples, Jesus said]: "Lazarus is dead, and for your sake I am glad I was not there, so that you may *believe*."

11:25–27 Jesus said to her [Martha]: "I am the resurrection and the life. He who *believes* in me will live, even though he dies; and whoever lives and *believes* in me will never die. Do you *believe* this?" "Yes, Lord," she told him, "I *believe* that you are the Christ, the Son of God, who was to come into the world."

11:40   Then Jesus said [to Martha]: "Did I not tell you that if you *believed*, you would see the glory of God?"

11:42   [Jesus prayed to the Father]: "I knew that you always hear me, but I said this for the benefit of the people standing here, that they may *believe* that you sent me."

11:48   [The Pharisees and the chief priests said to the Sanhedrin]: "If we let him go on like this, everyone will *believe* in him, and then the Romans will come and take away both our place and our nation."

John: Passage:

12:37–39 "Even after Jesus had done all these miraculous signs in their presence, they still would not *believe* in him. This was to fulfill the word of Isaiah the prophet: "Lord, who has *believed* our message and to whom has the arm of the Lord been revealed?" …For this reason they could not *believe*, because, as Isaiah says elsewhere: "He has blinded their eyes and deadened their hearts…"

12:42 "Yet at the same time many even among the leaders *believed* in him. But because of the Pharisees, they would not confess their faith for fear they would be put out of the synagogue. For they loved praise from men more than praise from God."

12:44, 46 Then Jesus cried out, "When a man *believes* in me, he does not *believe* in me only, but in the one who sent me." … "I have come into the world as a light, so that no one who *believes* in me should stay in darkness."

13:19 [Jesus said to his disciples prior to His betrayal]: "I am telling you now before it happens, so that when it does happen you will *believe* that I am He."

John: Passage:

14:10–11   [Jesus said to Phillip]: "Don't you *believe* that I am
           in the Father, and that the Father is in me? The
           words I say to you are not just my own. Rather, it
           is the Father living in me who is doing his work.
           Believe me when I say that I am in the Father
           and the Father is in me, or at least *believe* on the
           evidence of the miracles themselves."

14:29   [Jesus said to his disciples about the crucifixion]:
           "I have told you now before it happens, so that
           when it does happen you will *believe*."

16:8–9   [Jesus speaking to the disciples about the Holy
           Spirit]: "When he comes, he will convict the world
           of guilt in regard to sin and righteousness and judg-
           ment; in regard to sin, because men do not *believe*
           in me..."

16:27   [Jesus said to the disciples]: "No, the Father himself
           loves you because you have loved me and have
           believed that I came from God. I came from the
           Father and entered the world; now I am leaving the
           world and going back to the Father."

16:30–31   [Jesus said to his disciples]: "You *believe* at last."
           Jesus answered. "But a time is coming, and has
           come, when you will be scattered, each to his own
           home. You will leave me all alone. Yet I am not
           alone, for my Father is with me."

John: Passage:

17:8   [Jesus in prayer to the Father]: "For I gave them the words you gave me and they accepted them. They knew with certainty that I came from you and they *believed* that you sent me."

17:20–21   [Jesus prayed to the Father]: "My prayer is not for them [the disciples] alone. I pray also for those who will *believe* in me through their message, that all of them may be one, Father, just as you are in me and I am in you."

19:35   "The man [John] who saw it has given testimony, and his testimony is true. He knows that he tells the truth, and he testifies so that you also may *believe*."

20:8   "Finally, the other disciple [John] who had reached the tomb first, also went inside. He saw and *believed*."

20:25   So the other disciple [John] told him [Thomas], "We have seen the Lord." But he [Thomas] said to them, "Unless I see the nail marks in his hands and put my finger where the nails were, and put my hand into his side, I will not *believe* it."

John: Passage:

20:27–29   [Jesus said to the disciples]: "Peace be with you."
           Then he said to Thomas, "Put your finger here;
           see my hands. Reach out your hand and put it into
           my side. Stop doubting and **believe**." Thomas
           said to him, "My Lord and my God!" Then Jesus
           told him, "Because you have seen me, you have
           believed; blessed are those who have not seen and
           yet have **believed**."

20:31   [John said to the readers]: "But these matters are
           written that you may **believe** that Jesus is the
           Christ, the Son of God, and that by **believing** you
           may have life in his name."

Believe in His Name

Since the beginning of time, people have given great value and significance to a man's name. A man's name reveals his cultural background, his family within that culture, his character for honesty, his reputation among his peers and a variety of other characteristics. A man's good name should be valued above all else.

It is not surprising that man should want to know what name to call God. In Exodus 3, Moses meets God and has the following conversation:

"The Lord said, 'I have indeed seen the misery of my people in Egypt. I have heard them crying out because of their slave drivers, and I am concerned about their suffering. So I have come down to rescue them from the hand of the Egyptians and to bring them up out of that land into a good and spacious land, a land of milk and honey-- the home of the Canaanites, Hittites, Amorites, Perizzites, Hivites and Jebusites. And now the cry of the Israelites has reached me, and I have seen the way the Egyptians are oppressing them. So now, go. I am sending you to Pharaoh to bring my people the Israelites out of Egypt.'

"But Moses said to God: 'Who am I, that I should go to Pharaoh and bring the Israelites out of Egypt?'

"And God said: 'I will be with you. And this will be the sign to you that it is I who have sent you: When you have brought the people out of Egypt, you will worship God on the mountain.'

"Moses said to God, 'Suppose I go to the Israelites and say to them, "The God of your fathers has sent me to you," and they ask me, "What is his name?" Then what shall I tell them?'

"God said to Moses, "I AM WHO I AM." This is what you are to say to the Israelites: I AM has sent me to you." Exodus 3:7–14

We are told to pray in the name of Jesus, but what name shall we use? There are fifty-three different names for Jesus in the Gospel of John alone. Together, they capture most of the characteristics of Jesus, but Jesus is referred to by many other names throughout both the Old and New Testaments. When praying to Jesus, any of His many names will work. The following are the names for Jesus as found in John:

John:	Name for Jesus:
6:51	Bread
6:33	Bread of God
6:35; 6:48	Bread of Life
6:41; 6:58	Bread that came down from Heaven
3:29	Bridegroom
1:4; 4:29; 7:26, 41; 11:27	Christ
20:30	Christ, the
15:13–15	Friend

John:	Name for Jesus:
10:9	Gate
10:7	Gate for the sheep
10:36; 11:4	God's Son
10:11	Good Shepherd
8:58	I am
13:19	I am He
10:30	I and the Father are One
6:69	Holy One of God
5:45; 18:5, 8	Jesus of Nazareth
1:17	Jerusalem
5:30	Judge
18:37–39; 19:3, 19	King of the Jews
5:49; 12:13	King of Israel
1:29	Lamb of God
11:25; 14:6 1:7; 3:19–20	Life, the
2:35–38; 12:46	Light
8:12	Light of life
8:12; 9:5	Light of the world
6:51	Living bread
4:10	Living water

John:	Name for Jesus:
6:68: 9:38; 11:3, 12, 21, 27, 32, 34, 12:39, 41; 13:6, 9, 13–14, 13:25, 36, 37; 14:5	Lord
1:41; 4:25–26	Messiah
3:16, 18	One and Only Son
5:38	One He Sent
3:34	One whom God has sent
6:14; 7:40	Prophet
1:38, 49; 3:2, 4:31; 6:25: 9:1	Rabbi
20:16	Rabboni
11:25	Resurrection
3:35–36; 6:40; 8:36	Son
1:34; 49; 5:25; 1:27; 19:7; 20:30	Son of God
5:1, 13–14, 27; 6:27, 52; 8:27; 9:35; 12:23, 34; 13:31	Son of Man
4:36	Sower
4:42	Savior of the World

John:	Name for Jesus:
8:4; 11:28; 13:13–14; 20:10	Teacher
2:21	Temple
1:9	True light
15:1	True vine
14:6	Truth, the
15:5	Vine
14:6	Way, the
1:1	Word
1:14	Word became flesh

The ancient fascination with the names of God continues even today. For a learned treatise on this subject, see *All the Divine Names and Titles in the Bible* by Henry Lockerby. This is Volume 4 of a multi-volume set called the "All" series. This book was published by Zondervan Publishing (1975).

For a more readable book on the subject of the names of Jesus, see *He Shall be Called: The 150 Names of Jesus and What They Mean to You,* by Robert J. Morgan, published by Time Warner Books Group (2005).

PART III:

WHAT OTHERS PROFESS TO BELIEVE

Lessons from
50 Spiritual Classics

Timeless Wisdom from 50 Great Books of
Inner Discovery, Enlightenment and Purpose
Edited by Tom Butler-Bowdon (MJF Books, 2005)

The following is a summary of some of the ideas contained in
the *50 Spiritual Classics*:

We are not an accident of science.
We were created, so there must be a Creator.
Since we were created, we must have a purpose and reason
to be.

We are spiritual beings.
We exist to glorify the Creator.
We seek spiritual oneness with the Creator.

Our purpose is to seek God with our whole being.
Our purpose is to praise God with all we are.
Our purpose is to embrace God's presence at all things.

Giving thanks is freeing and fulfilling.
Peace comes with believing God is in all things.
Poise means accepting God's blessings.

The physical world is ordered according to the laws of nature.
The political world is ordered according to the rule of law.
The spiritual world is ordered according to the will of God.

There are no ordinary moments.
Every moment is spiritual.
Each moment is pregnant with possibilities.

Religious beliefs and spiritual truths are different.
Religion consists of rules, beliefs and practices.
Spiritual awaking results from personal experiences.

Western religions celebrate materialism and power.
Individual achievement gives voice to pride and pleasure.
Spiritual secrets are not found in what is seen, touched or heard.

Eastern mysticism seeks meaning from the unseen.
Solitude and silence enhance a spiritual quest for the Creator.
Self-surrender reveals the mystery of peace and joy.

Learning and knowledge do not equal Truth.
Seeking God brings peace.
The one true path to God is Jesus.

Love is the basic principle of all life.
Peace is experienced only through oneness with God.
Illumination arrives from the spiritual silence of solitude.

Modern physics believes that the physical world is explainable.
Events happen because of cause and effect.
All causes have effects. All effects have causes.

Modern physics claims that the past can be replicated.
Patterns follow rules and are not random.
Deviations can be explained.

Mysticism teaches that all things consist of energy.
Energy forces are perpetually in motion.
Energy particles are constantly colliding, resulting in random events.

Mysticism explains random acts as spiritual events.
Signs and symbols reveal the mystery of the spiritual.
Miracles happen through divine intervention.

I am not in control. God is.
Every moment is a miracle.
The present is a gift from the Creator.

There are no coincidences.
Seemingly random events are not random.
Divine appointments connect past, present and future.

No comparison with others advances the truth.
No criticism of others elevates your status.
No compliment of others goes unrewarded.

Each moment is a miracle.
Each moment contains a miracle.
Living in the moment defines the future.

Pursuing God in all things transforms the bad and confirms the good.
Seeking God always results in finding God.
Searching for God's presence in all things turns all things into joy.

Security is illusory.

Peace comes from the absence of things, not the abundance of things.

Things are not the goal. God is.

Mercy is what God gives when we deserve judgment.

Grace is what God gives when we deserve punishment.

Life is what God gives when death is all around us.

Lessons from Ecclesiastes

Solomon, the author of Ecclesiastes, is often referred to as the Teacher and is regarded by history as the world's richest and smartest man. He wrote the Proverbs during his early life to provide guidance to others on how to lead a moral and significant life, a life of wisdom and truth. But after searching for a life of significance and satisfaction, even with all his abundance, Solomon never found peace or satisfaction of joy through his possessions, power or influence. In fact, all of the things that man seeks to achieve through his own efforts, all those things we pursue to make a living, are illusive, not fulfilling and are not what we hope them to be. They are all "meaningless and chasing after the wind," according to Solomon.

Here are some examples of what man pursues in the hope of having success, but which, Solomon concludes, are "meaningless" and "chasing after the wind:"

Ecc:	Man's Goal:
1:4	Achievement
1:14; 12:8	All things
2:2-7	Cattle
5:7	Dreaming
1:14: 3:19 1:2; 2:11;	Enlightenment

Ecc:	Man's Goal:
11:8; 12:8	Everything
2:2-7	Homes
6:1	Honor
1:1	Knowledge
4:4	Labor
2:2-7	Laughter
9:9	Life
5:10	Money
1:14	Possessions
8:14	Righteousness
2:2-7	Slaves
2:2-7	Treasures
1:11; 1:17	Understanding
11:10	Vigor
2:2-7	Vineyards
5:10	Wealth
1:11; 1:17	Wisdom
11:10	Youth

The Teacher also says that life is NOT about:

Acquisitions, achievements or awards.

Blessings, blame or burdens.

Comfort, courage or crowns.

Deeds, decency or delights.

Endurance, evidence or existence.

Fruit, fellowship or forgiveness.

Grace, goodness or giving.

Happiness, honors or humility.

Image, income or interests.

Justice, judgment or joy.

Kindness, kinship or knowledge.

Land, labor or law.

Money, mountains or miracles.

Names, needs or neighbors.

Origins, obligations or oaths.

Past, present or prominence.

Powers, prestige or position.

Questions, qualities or quiet.

Resolve, rewards or rights.

Silver, struggles or success.

Tasks, tests or triumphs.

Urges, usefulness or understanding.

Valley, vale or value.

Wages, want or wealth.

Wishes, will or wisdom.

Experience, expectancies or the extraordinary.

External, excellence or exhortations.

Yesterday, yearning or yoke.

Zeal, zealots or Zion.

CONCLUSION FROM THE TEACHER:

"Now all has been heard; here is the conclusion of the matter: **Fear God and keep his commandments, for this is the whole duty of man**. For God will bring every deed into judgment, including every hidden thing, whether good or evil." Ecclesiastes 12:13-14

This I Believe Project

The _This I Believe Project_ was a weekly radio program begun by Edward R. Morrow in the 1950s. He asked celebrities and ordinary people, "What do you believe?" _This I Believe_ is also a recently published book in which Jay Allison and Dan Gediman of National Public Radio compiled and edited the statements of belief of many of those who appeared on the Morrow program. The following is a summary of what some people responded when asked, "What do you believe?"

[The term "I" in the selections below does not refer to the author of this book. Instead, the "I" refers to a participant in the _This I Believe Project_.]

I believe that truth is not relative. . . though it may be elusive or hidden. People may wish to disregard it. But there is such a thing as truth. . . What really matters is the pursuit of truth.

I believe that the journey is all, not the goal.

I believe in the pursuit and the act. One without the other is self-indulgence. Aim for truth without accusation, patriotism without political comment, faith beyond religious dogma.

I believe that beliefs are choices. No one has authority over your personal beliefs.

I believe that we should practice humility and forgiveness, empathy and equality, caring and compassion.

I believe that I am free to be whomever I choose to be.

I believe that you only have what you give away...knowledge, experience, talent and love.

I believe in remembering those that came before.

I believe in people. I feel, love, need and respect others.

I believe that man's noblest endowment is his capacity to change.

I believe that life is a journey. . . You make the trip by faith: Words don't count; it's not what I say but what I do that counts.

I believe that no job is more important than being a parent.

I believe that my own self-esteem reflects my ability to make a difference for others.

I believe that we depend on others.

I believe that the fabric of my life is woven with gratitude and humility; there is strength and freedom in surrender.

I believe that the guiding light of my life is the Holy Spirit, the still small voice within me.

I believe that the purpose of my daily walk is just to listen and care.

I believe that prayer is more about what I hear than what I say.

I believe that spiritual truth is not about religion as much as Spirit. "Be still and know that I am God."

The holy core of my life is exposed during the elusive whispers between me and God.

I believe, "If I die, it will be glory. If I live, it will be grace."

I believe in faith greater than man, faith in the One Creator, Giver of Life, the Omnipotent One.

I believe that man is on a long journey to be free from a need for something bigger than self.

I believe a doubting mind is both a blessing and a curse.

I believe in now, so I spend time engaged in the present. "Wherever you are, be there."

I believe in the free and responsible development of the individual, so that he may serve mankind.

I believe in naming things, breaking through taboos, challenging current beliefs.

I believe in taking personal responsibility to make a positive impact on society through an unquenchable thirst for knowledge and truth, through striving for excellence, through service to mankind.

I believe in God, not the cosmic-intangible-Spirit-in-the-sky-kind-of-God, but the God who embraced me when daddy disappeared. I have come to know Abba as my Father.

I believe in the power of intelligence and creativity to make the world a better place.

I believe in families, not just those that are connected by blood, but also those that are connected when no one else will show up.

I believe in the connection between a stranger when he reaches out to help others.

I believe in learning by practice and performance over and over again and in the cultivation of just being.

I believe in the ability to see beautiful precise pictures, even though I am bipolar.

I believe in disrupting my comfort zone, challenging myself with interesting people.

I believe in the process of going from confusion to under-standing, from uncertainty to discovery.

I believe in preferring to listen rather than to speak, to inquire and not to crusade.

I believe in the power of being there, in the power of presence, in "being there with."

I believe in imagining life and trying to live it.

I believe in being happy, in the goodness of man and in the belief that good will triumph over evil.

I believe we are not alone, that others have been here before us and they are still here.

I believe that everything is connected dynamically at the intimate level, in the sacredness of life.

I believe in my neighbors. I know their faults, and I know that their virtues far outweigh their faults.

I believe in the honesty, insatiable curiosity, unlimited courage and noble essential decency of my neighbor.

I believe that there is more good than evil, more of those who create than those who destroy, more who love than hate. The nectar of life is sweet only when it is shared with others.

I believe that curiosity, wonder and passion are defining qualities of imaginative minds and great teachers.

I believe that I am not religious, but I am spiritual.

I believe in faith wrought into life apart from creed or dogma. By faith, I mean a vision of what is good and enthusiastic, the dynamic power that breaks the chain of the routine. Faith is a state of mind not soon disheartened.

I believe in the reverence for beauty and preciousness of the earth.

I believe that freedom is contagious. The only difference between the darkness of North Korea and the lights of South Korea is the government that rules them.

I believe that love is primal. It is comprised of compassion, care, security and a leap of faith. I believe in the power of love to transform.

I believe in the power of the unknown. I believe in the exhilaration of standing at the boundary between the known and the unknown.

I believe that time is the supreme, most useful gift...without a beginning or end, birth or death, there is no time.

I believe in the power of friendship, which grows out of love and true humility. It is the most important thing in life.

I believe in honor, faith, truth and integrity.

I believe in the absolute and unlimited liberty of reading.

I believe in truth and in the pursuit of truth.

I believe in the rule of law. It is probably the single greatest achievement of our society. It is our bulwark against both mob rule and overwhelming power of the modern state. It is simultaneously wonderfully strong and precariously fragile.

I believe a little outrage can go a long way.

I believe in empathy. I believe in the kind of empathy that is created through imagination and through intimate, personal relationships.

I believe in poetry as a way of surviving the emotional chaos, spiritual confusion and traumatic events that come with being alive.

I believe that America is humanity's best opportunity to make God's wish that we come to know one another a reality.

I believe in the 50% theory. Half the time things are better than normal; the other half they are worse.

I believe in America and the generosity of its people. Our greatest strength is our openness and our welcoming nature.

I believe in the struggle to balance the clanging, colliding rights of others.

I believe that there is more to life than life. That's why there are flowers on the graves.

I believe that tomorrow will be better than today.

I believe that each of us has a chance, not a guarantee. I believe that what was done for me God sustained. I believe in man's integrity and in the goodness of a free society. I believe that there is progress, even when it comes very slowly.

I believe that everyone is obligated to do his very best.

I believe in cultivating hidden talents, buried and unrelated to what we do for a living.

I believe in humility. I believe that the deadliest sin is pride.

I believe that freedom comes the hard way, by ceaseless groping, toil, struggle, even by fiery trial and agony.

I believe that we must be bridge builders for those who come after us.

I believe that the sound of jazz is the laughter of God, and I believe that if you keep moving forward, you'll get there.

I believe in barbecue, as soul food and comfort and health food, as a cuisine of both solace and celebration. I believe that like sunshine and great sex, no day is a bad day that has barbecue in it.

I believe in politics. Politics is basically the peaceable resolution of conflict among legitimate competing interests. Compromises that are both wise and just are crafted through politics.

Moderation is one of the virtues I most believe in. I also believe in kindness, generosity, steadfastness and courage. I believe that good depends not on things but on the use we make of things. I fear passionate faith and immoderate zeal.

I believe that I was born luckier than most; therefore, I was born more obligated than most.

I believe in nature and nurture, heredity and society. I believe that we have no idea what might be possible for us on this earth.

I believe in life, in treasuring it as a mystery that can never be truly understood, as a sanctity that should never be destroyed. I believe in liberty. I believe in free speech, the right to offend, the pursuit of happiness.

I believe in rituals and ceremonies and traditions.
They give meaning and texture to the purpose of culture.

I believe that what matters most is not one's knowledge and skill, but one's friendships and relationships with others.

I believe that love is what gives life meaning and purpose.

I believe in the American experiment, and I believe that religious faith will continue to be an essential part of being human.

I believe in the power of inspiration, in the mysterious gift of creation.

I believe that the highest quality of life is full of art and creative expression.

I believe in the rule of law, in the sense of mutual obligation.

I believe that ordinary people do extraordinary things, that truth is told in the actions we take.

PART IV:

WHAT I BELIEVE AS A RESULT OF PERSONAL EXPERIENCES

A PERSONAL TESTIMONY: 1997

Most of you know me as a lawyer, as the father of two terrific children and as a member of First United Methodist Church in Tulsa active in church finance and administrative matters. My opportunities to serve the church came, because I volunteered for one project. In late 1981, Dr. Thomas announced from the pulpit that the church planned to refinance the bank indebtedness incurred for the construction of the new children's wing by selling church bonds. After the service, I volunteered to help. The next day, Dr. Thomas appointed me special counsel to the church for the church bond offering. In February 1982 the church sold $2,000,000 in church bonds to church members. The bonds fixed the interest rate, extended the maturity and allowed the church certainty in budgeting. Because I took the first step to volunteer, I have been blessed with many opportunities to serve.

This is the rest of the story. There are three major pillars in my life: my family, my job and my relationship with God. These three priorities define who I am, what I stand for and why I do what I have done. Achieving balance has proven to be quite difficult at times There are always competing demands on my time that threaten to disrupt the balance. Recently, various events have shaken the very foundation of my life.

Fired

For six years immediately prior to June 30, 1992, I was a named partner in an excellent law firm in Tulsa. My partners were my friends. We had no serious disagreements. We had common objectives and common goals. But on June 30, 1992, without warning or explanation, I was asked to leave the partnership. When I asked why, the answer was, "We're not going to tell you." For five of the six years of our partnership, I had been instrumental in securing more new clients which produced more revenue for the firm than any other lawyer. Being asked to leave the firm made no sense to me. I now believe that God was at work, giving me a wakeup call. One of the main pillars in my life, my job, was knocked out from under me without warning or explanation.

Two weeks later, Judge Cook, the senior trial judge on the federal bench in Tulsa, announced his decision to take senior status, leaving a vacancy in that position. Since law school, I have believed that I would one day be a federal judge. I thought Judge Cook's decision was the explanation for my being fired. Cautiously, I spent weeks praying over whether or not I should submit my name to seek the nomination to fill the vacancy. I spent the next two and a half months pursuing that federal judgeship. I honestly believed that God wanted me to be a federal judge. Being confirmed would turn the devastation of being fired into a life time dream realized.

Forgotten

The process of selecting a federal judge is extremely political and usually very secret. The custom is that the President nominates the person named by the senior U.S. senator of the same political party as the President from the state where the judgeship is open. There was no practical or logical reason why I thought I would receive the nomination, since I was not a high profile political supporter or friend of Senator Nickles and since it had been a long time since I had even tried a case in federal court (and that was in Texas).

The chairman of the selection committee was a high school friend and former partner of mine at Hall Estill. My mentor throughout college and law school and a former federal judge was appointed a member of the selection committee. Many prominent Tulsans actively supported my selection. The committee interviewed forty-five candidates and selected three names to submit to Senator Nickles. My name was not on the short list. I felt forgotten, and I believed that I had let God down. How silly!

As a footnote, the person selected by Senator Nickles and nominated by President Bush was a close personal friend of Senator Nickles but was never even voted upon by the Senate Judiciary Committee, because President Bush was not re-elected. God was at work protecting me from that turmoil, but I did not know it at the time.

Frozen Out

In February 1993, after almost twenty-five years of marriage, I reached the conclusion that my marriage was no marriage at all, and there was not much that I could do about it. Claudia and I have the two greatest children in the world. Laura and Kipp became our lives. I was a terrific father. I set out to be the perfect dad. If there is a fault in this, I probably made my family my God. I worshipped my family. I defined myself by describing them. If Laura or Kipp were doing something, I was there. They love me, and I love them unconditionally. Claudia was an excellent mother, but except for the kids' activities, Claudia and I did not participate together in anything. We shared no contact, communication or affection. Our interests, our desires and our lives went different directions.

My family was crumbling out from under me, but I was unable to figure out what to do to make it work. I felt Claudia did not care for me, did not love me, did not want me around and would be happier without me there. I did not make her happy, and everything I tried to do to make her happy was turned against me. I was constantly criticized, blamed for everything that went wrong, even ridiculed and finally I was just ignored. When I could not stand it any longer, I moved out of the house.

Frightened

I got sick. I contracted an unexplained infection, an unidentified parasite and an unidentified virus all at the same time. Antibiotics did not work, and other medication did not help. The result was serious depression. Somehow, I continued to work, but most of the work was also depressing. Again, I thought I had let God, my wife and my family down. I got frightened. I prayed earnestly for a solution. I am a problem solver in business and in law. I could help solve everybody else's problems, but I could not figure out how to solve my own.

First Men

In early 1994, while attending a church executive committee meeting, I joked with Joanne Stafford, president of the local United Methodist Women, "Why is there a woman on the executive committee representing the United Methodist Women when there is no man representing United Methodist Men? Equal is equal, after all." Joanne challenged me to start a men's ministry program in the church.

Within six weeks, eleven other men approached Dr. Buskirk, our senior pastor, with the idea of starting a men's ministry program. None of us knew each other, and no one knew what shape or form the men's ministry program should take. After three months of brainstorming, we decided that First Men should not focus on "bowling, banquets or Bar-B-Qs." Rather, we wanted something substantive, not social. We decided to ask prominent businessmen to tell how their faith makes a difference in their daily lives.

In October 1995, First Men chartered two buses to go to Promise Keepers in Dallas. I did not want to go, and I did not want First Men to get lost as a local Promise Keeper chapter. When Dub Ambrose, our leader, asked me to be a bus captain,

I agreed to go, but I did so for all the wrong reasons. I was intellectually curious. I wanted to know how PK could feed 75,000 men lunch in twenty-five minutes. I could not imagine sitting in a stadium on a Friday night for four hours with no women present and no game to watch. I definitely could not believe that 75,000 men would voluntarily sit through hours of sermons all day Saturday too. The Dallas Promise Keepers' conference changed my life.

Fired Up

Friday evening, we saw James Ryle, Coach McCartney's pastor, throw a deflated football around Texas Stadium and tell his heart wrenching story of being imprisoned in a jail built by his father. Then Tony Evans gave the best and clearest description of discipleship I have ever heard. He ended by describing the final scene in *Rocky IV*, where Mickey, Rocky's old boxing coach, who had died but came back to Rocky in a dream, told Rocky to: "Get up, get up, you bum, 'Cause Mickey loves you!" But for Tony Evans, it was: "Get up, get up, you bums, 'Cause Jesus loves you!" Like the other 75,000 men there, I got up and worshipped Jesus with song and praise. It was a magical time. The next morning, I was the first one back in Texas Stadium. I was exhilarated and excited and wanted more.

Most of the 130 First Men were sitting together at the far end of the Texas Stadium on the second level directly opposite the platform. There were two vacant seats next to me, because Dub Ambrose and his son left temporarily to get a drink. Two young men sat in Dub's seats. I explained the situation, but they said that they were just there for a little while. They were off duty members of the Dallas Police Department. They had heard about Promise Keepers, and they were curious.

At the end of his presentation, Jack Hayford asked us to get in groups of four or five men and to pray for each other. The two young Dallas policemen joined our prayer group. I asked John, "What's bothering you?" He said, "Man, my dad is a minister, and he did something really bad. I have not been able to go back to my church ever since." I said, "John, you need to forgive your dad." John began to cry. The five of us prayed. That was the first time I had ever prayed directly for someone else in their presence. John asked God to forgive his father, and John did forgive his father right before our eyes. John was freed from his grief, guilt and embarrassment. He went away from us that morning a new person, forgiven and free.

Forgiven and Free

I left Promise Keepers in Dallas 1995 a different man too, a committed Christian, also forgiven and free, just like John. Up to that point in my life, I had been a passive Christian. Although I was active in church committees, I was not on fire for Christ. I learned three lessons:

Lesson One: I had to be fired from an all consuming job to regain humility. I had to be forgotten in the federal court nomination process to realize that God was in charge, not me. I had to be broken to become bold.

Lesson Two: I had to volunteer to help with the church bond drive before God could use me for greater purposes. I had to reach up to Him, so that He could lift me up to be where He is. God does not always use the most qualified, but He always qualifies the most available.

Lesson Three: I had to surrender myself and my pride, so that He could set me free to be His instrument.

In summary, I believe:

- I was fired, so that I would be humbled before God.

- I was forgotten, so that I might show obedience to God.

- I was frozen out of my family, so that I would focus on God.

- I was frightened, so that I might know faith in God.

- I was forgiven and freed, so that I could be used for God's purposes.

The fires of this process have often been painful. I am still a work in process. But those trials have purified, refined and strengthened me. They were necessary for me to break through the walls of self and pride in order to surrender more to Him. I am His; and I thank God for the mysterious, incomprehensible, unimaginable, unbelievable gift of His grace. To God Be the Glory!

MY JOURNEY OF FAITH: 2006

My journey began on August 21, 1943 at St. John's Hospital in Tulsa. I was baptized on October 31, 1943 at First Lutheran Church in Tulsa. Baseball, Boy Scouts and church were my priorities in my early years. In 1955, my brother, Phil. and I were the third and fourth Boy Scouts in Oklahoma to earn the *Pro Deo et Patria*, the Lutheran God and Country Award. We were both Eagle Scouts and Brotherhood Members of Order of the Arrow. I was confirmed at First Lutheran Church in May 1956 after two years of study every Saturday morning. The first book report I gave at Edison High School was on *Here I Stand* by Roland Bainton, the definitive biography of Martin Luther.

At KU, I regularly attended church and occasionally attended Campus Crusade for Christ meetings. After graduation from KU Law School in 1968, I entered active military service and taught an adult Sunday school class at Ft. Lewis, Washington, my first duty station as an Army lawyer. Following almost three years in Germany and after I earned a Master of Laws Degree from Harvard in 1973, my wife, Claudia, and I settled in Dallas, where our two children, Laura and Kipp, were born and baptized at the Prestonwood Presbyterian Church in Dallas.

We returned to Tulsa in 1980 and joined First Methodist Church at the Christmas morning service, where Dr. L. D. Thomas, a lawyer turned minister, was the senior pastor. My active involvement at First Methodist began in the fall of 1981 when I volunteered to help in a church bond program to refinance the bank debt incurred to build the children's addition. Dr. Thomas appointed me special counsel to the church and a member of the finance committee. Within four months, the church completed a $2,000,000 church bond program. Later, I wrote *A Practical Guide to Church Bond Financing* to help other churches finance church expansions with a bond financing program. I have since served First Methodist in many leadership positions. I have learned a lot about churches and a lot about God, but I did not know Jesus in an intimate and personal way until 1995.

By the early1990s, I had achieved some success as a business lawyer and was a named partner in a prominent downtown Tulsa law firm. My priorities in life were family first, job next and church last. My core values focused on family, friends and faith. In June 1992, things started falling apart. Without warning or explanation, I was fired from my law firm, even though my clients paid more fees to the firm than the clients of any other partner for five of the six years I was in the firm and even though I was responsible for more new clients than any other partner. After leaving the firm, I believed that I would be appointed to the federal bench. I was wrong. My twenty-five year marriage began to sour. I became frightened and depressed. My faith was challenged at my very core.

In 1994, I joined eleven other men in urging Dr. James Buskirk, our Senior Pastor, to create a men's ministry program. I soon discovered that most men today are intensely competitive, task oriented, emotionally lonely, highly individualistic, essentially friendless and spiritually hungry. First Men began meeting monthly to hear how faith in God makes a difference in the daily lives of successful businessmen and community leaders. Many of their testimonies became building blocks in my journey of faith. First Men continues today to provide encouragement to men in their spiritual journey to find Jesus.

In late October 1995, First Men chartered two buses to Dallas for a Promise Keepers conference. I did not want to go, but I agreed to go when I was asked to be the bus captain for one of the buses. Intellectually, I was curious to see if men would fill a stadium for four hours of worship on Friday evening without a game involved or women to watch and then come back for more all day Saturday. I also could not believe that 75,000 men could be fed lunch in twenty-five minutes. What happened at Promise Keepers changed my life.

The conference opened with awesome praise and worship music like I had never heard. We first heard the heart wrenching testimony of James Ryle, Coach Bill McCartney's pastor, tell how he was jailed in a prison his father had built. Dr. Tony Evans of Dallas then told how a messed up man causes a messed up family, a messed up neighborhood and a messed up nation. To have a better nation, a better neighborhood and a better family, it all starts by becoming better men. Dr. Evans concluded by describing a scene from the movie, *Rocky IV*. When Rocky was down and almost out, his old coach, Mickey, who had died, came to tell him in a vision, urging Rocky to: "Get up, get up, you bum! 'Cause Mickey loves you." But Dr. Evans said instead, "Get up, get up, you bums! 'Cause Jesus loves you." I was hooked. The messages and music in Dallas spoke to me in a deep and personal way.

When I returned to Tulsa, I ordered the speaker tapes from the Dallas Promise Keepers event to share with the men of First Methodist and others. On January 4, 1996 and for more than eight years thereafter, I lead a men's Power Lunch every Thursday where we watched a Promise Keepers video, sang some praise and worship songs, ate some pizza and prayed for the men that came. Many men from various denominations, including many pastors, were blessed by Jesus at these lunches.

In May 1999, our daughter, Laura, graduated from Emory University Law School in Atlanta, and our son, Kipp, graduated from Boston College. As part of my graduation gift to them, I compiled a collection of stories from my life experiences, especially the funny war stories from some of my trials as a lawyer in the Army. That compilation was entitled, *Angels All Around.* By looking back, I discovered that God's angels had always been protecting me from myself, even when I did not know it. God uses our brokenness to make us bold for Him.

My excitement about Jesus has increased since my first Promise Keepers experience. I have continued to attend national and local Promise Keepers events. I have read widely about how Jesus makes all the difference, especially in the lives of men in the marketplace who surrender to His call. I began to take my daily devotional time more seriously. After reading several different devotionals, I discovered that I needed a more disciplined approach to my devotional time. So I divided the Psalms into 366 days, and I wrote down my reflections and my thoughts on a daily basis. The beauty of the Psalms, the sweep of emotions confronted by the Psalms and my search for meaning, purpose and significance through the Psalms resulted in *Seeking God's Heart: A Devotional Journey through the Psalms* (2004), and *A Treasury of Truth and Wisdom* (2007*)*, a collection of Biblically-based aphorisms intended to encourage the reader to move from success to significance.

My journey has not always been smooth, successful or pleasant. The trials and difficulties have refined and strengthened me. I continue to be a work in progress, consciously seeking God's presence. I have learned that surrendering to God's will is the key to success, that seeking God's heart is the key to significance and that striving to be in God's presence is the key to experiencing His peace and His joy. To God be the glory!

This article appears at Page 112 of *Journey: Tulsa's Century of Christian Faith, Leadership and Influence*, by Tom McCloud and Tara Lynn Thompson, published by McCloud Media (2006).

DIVINE MOMENTS: 2009

Do you believe in accidents? Do you believe in coincidences? Do you believe that seemingly random occurrences are really "divine moments" orchestrated by God Himself?" I do.

In May 1999, our daughter, Laura, was preparing to graduate from Emory Law School in Atlanta. Laura was also planning her wedding on Saturday, the weekend before our son, Kipp, was to graduate from Boston College the following Monday. In anticipation of those events, I wrote *Angels All Around*, a collection of stories about my early years and some of the funny things that I experienced while practicing law, especially while I was a Captain in the Army.

While writing *Angels*, I discovered how God had protected me, provided for me, selected me, used me and prepared me at every critical moment of my life. I learned three fundamental truths:

1. God is present in my life, even when I do not acknowledge Him and even when I reject Him.

2. God uses people as messengers to change lives. Some people know the effect they have on others, but many have no clue how they have changed another person's life.

3. Defining moments can become divine moments if we are open to the influences of God's messengers.

Summer, 1961: Ed Strong

I had just graduated from Edison High School in Tulsa and was excited about becoming a freshman at the University of Kansas. On an ordinary day during the summer before leaving for Lawrence, I enjoyed my annual lunch with my Dad. He was very proud of his three boys, and once a year he invited each of us separately to have lunch with him. It was a special occasion for me and my brothers. We always went to lunch at a Tulsa landmark, Nelson's Buffeteria, where we always ordered chicken fried steak, green beans, mashed potatoes with cream gravy and a piece of banana cream pie.

On our way to lunch, Dad and I met Ed Strong, who worked with my father at Amerada Petroleum and a man I knew as Scout Master of Troop 37 long after I finished Scouts. Mr. Strong was also a Colonel in the Army Reserves. He asked me about school and then said: "Are you going to sign up for ROTC?" No one in my immediate family had been in the military, and the thought of being in ROTC had never occurred to me. I innocently asked, "Why should I do that?" He responded: "Because it will be an easy A."

This was the summer of 1961.The Korean conflict had been over for almost a decade. Peace prevailed, though the Cold War was in full swing. The thought of a war in Vietnam or anywhere else was inconceivable at the time to me. But I figured I would need all the A's I could get, so when I signed up for classes, I signed up for Army ROTC. This proved to be a defining moment for me.

I did get A's in ROTC my first two years at KU, and as a result, at the end of my sophomore year, I was given an award. I learned if I signed up to continue ROTC, I would receive $43/month while I was in school. I needed the money, so I signed up. Between my junior and senior years at KU, I attended ROTC summer camp at Ft. Riley, Kansas. There I learned about the Judge Advocate General Corps Excess Leave Program. If accepted, I would be assured that I would be able to finish law school before I served my tour of duty in the Army. This came with the price of an additional 6 months of obligated service for each year I was on "excess leave." The program also provided me with summer employment. I was obligated to return to active service when school was not in session for a week or more. That obligation was a blessing, since the money I made while on active status was needed for me to attend law school. I was accepted into the program. I received a regular (as opposed to reserve) commission as an Army Captain the same day I graduated from KU, and I immediately went on active duty. I reported to Ft. Sill, Oklahoma during the summers and while law school was not in session. I tried several special courts martial cases before graduating law school. I got paid while at Ft. Sill, but I did not get paid while I was attending classes at KU. Even so, I was on active duty, and my time in grade as an officer continued to count as if I were in an active status.

During 1965 to 1968, my law school years, every male student had to scramble to deal with the draft. Three months before I graduated from law school, three of my classmates were drafted when their local draft boards refused to grant further deferments for them to complete law school. Because I was in the Army, I did not have to worry about the draft. All I had to do was graduate and pass the bar exam. By the time

I graduated from law school, the United States had more than 650,000 active military personnel in Vietnam.

As a new JAGC officer, I attended the basic JAGC class held at the University of Virginia in Charlottesville, VA. My class consisted of 102 new Army lawyers, 77 of whom had graduated first in their law school class. The competition for these positions was fierce, but since I was already in the Army, I did not have to compete for the position. Captain John Freidenberger was my older brother's best friend in high school. He also made Captain's assignments for new JAGC officers. He asked me where I wanted to be assigned. I told him I wanted to go to the West Coast, either Ft. Lewis, Washington or Ft. Ord, California. Of the 102 new JAGC officers in my class, three were assigned to the West Coast. I was assigned to Ft. Lewis, Washington.

Upon arriving at Ft. Lewis, I reported to Colonel Dennis York, the post JAG. Within a couple minutes, Colonel York said, "You will be at Ft. Lewis approximately 1 year. You will either go to Vietnam or Europe from here. I have just returned from Germany, and I can help you get there if that is your desire." I said, "I want to go to Germany." A couple weeks later, John called and asked me where I wanted to be assigned in Germany and when. I told him that I wanted to be home for Christmas and to be assigned to the largest general jurisdiction in Europe. Eleven months later, I received orders for the US Army Europe Theater Army Support Command in Worms, Germany. We arrived in early February 1970, after spending Christmas at home and 3 weeks in an advanced government contracts class at the JAGC school in Charlottesville, VA.

While in Germany, I was able to prosecute many important cases, including a murder case. All general court martial convictions are automatically appealed to the US Court of Military Appeals in Washington, D.C. My law school roommate, John Toland, was assigned to defend on appeal the murderer I prosecuted. The case involved a homosexual assault by a young white soldier of a young black soldier. The black soldier responded by stabbing the white soldier forty-two times in the back. He was convicted of second degree murder and sentenced to twenty-five years. During sentencing, I presented several color photographs of the victim's back, showing a pin cushion appearance. John would later argue that the photos were unnecessarily graphic and warranted a reduction in sentencing.

During the appeal process, John informed me that the Army was proposing a reduction in force by granting early releases to officers who were accepted into graduate education programs. I applied for a Master of Laws program at Harvard, Yale, Michigan and Texas. I was accepted only by Harvard and was awarded a full tuition scholarship. I was permitted to resign my commission in early August 1972, in time for fall classes to begin in September.

Without the seemingly random comment by Ed Strong, the following events would not have happened:

I would not have enrolled in ROTC at KU.

I would not have gone to Ft. Riley, Kansas summer camp in 1967.

I would not have learned of the JAGC Excess Leave Program.

I would not have received $43/month during my junior and senior years at KU.

I would not have been able to finish law school without worrying about the draft.

I would not have been assigned to Ft. Lewis, Washington or Worms, Germany.

I would not have tried a murder case in Germany.

I would not have learned about the early release program in 1972.

I would not have gone to Harvard and earned a Master of Laws Degree.

November 1975: Unknown Angel

Another example of an angel sent by God to protect me from myself occurred in November 1975. I had been an associate with the Jackson Walker law firm in Dallas since June 1973. A number of events occurred that led me to question whether I was in the right place for me. I began to explore other options, including an exciting opportunity to become general counsel of an oil and gas company headquartered in Oklahoma City.

On Wednesday before Thanksgiving, I completed my second interview with the Oklahoma City company. The chance to be a top officer of a New York Stock Exchange listed company at age thirty-five, to be on the executive committee and to double my current compensation was very intriguing. I was offered the position, but I did not respond immediately, hoping for a few more stock options and other benefits. Claudia and I returned to Dallas, excited about the new opportunity. I decided over the weekend that I would call to accept the position at 10:00 a.m. on Monday morning.

At 9:30 a.m. Monday morning, I got a call from a person who would not identify himself other than to say that he was a former officer of the Oklahoma City company, that he knew I was interviewing there, that he knew something about me and that I should not take the job. I was shocked and curious. I asked why, and he said that he would not say. I asked for further information, and he referred me to the former general counsel, who worked in an office across the street. I had tried to find this former lawyer to ask why he left, but the company was reluctant to tell me anything other than he and his wife were Texans and missed home.

After several attempts, I convinced the former general counsel to let me take him to lunch. During lunch, he disclosed numerous financial and ethical issues that convinced me that I should not take the job. When I called the company to decline, they asked me why. I reported that I had visited with the former general counsel and what he told me was enough for me to decline, even if what he said was not entirely true.

Without the kindness of my unknown angel, calling to warn a stranger:

I would have accepted the offer from the Oklahoma City company.

I would have learned about its questionable financial dealings.

I would have been confronted with serious ethical challenges.

I would have had to resign without a prospect of future employment.

I would have been very unhappy.

December 1981: Dr. L. D. Thomas

Instead of moving to Oklahoma City, I accepted a job with a small Dallas firm, where I helped lawyer four successful public securities offerings in three years. I also participated in very important litigation with the objective of keeping Texas free from federal regulation of the electric utility industry.

In January 1980, I became a partner in that Dallas firm, but I was asked to move to Washington, D.C. for an expected three-plus year hearing before the Nuclear Regulatory Commission, which would litigate whether operating permits would be issued for two nuclear power plants in Texas. The question primarily involved anti-trust issues arising after the construction permits for the plants had been issued. I did not want to be away from my family, so I began to look for another opportunity.

I had interviewed for a general corporate law position with Hall Estill in Tulsa in January 1980. I received an offer on the spot, but I was so busy in Dallas I did not respond. In May my law school roommate, John Toland, was to be married in Miami, OK. He asked me to be in the wedding party. We went to the Friday night rehearsal and stayed with my mother in Tulsa Friday night. Saturday, we looked for houses in Tulsa and found the house of Claudia's dream. We made a low ball offer on Sunday and accepted the counter on Monday. I called Hall Estill and asked if the position was still open. It was. I accepted and stated to work on June 30, 1980.

The mortgage rates had been as high as 21% in late 1979, but they had dropped to 12.5% by June 1980. We sold our home in Dallas in 8 days for a substantial profit without a financing contingency and moved to Tulsa in less than 45 days. God and His angels were all over these events. They could not have happened without His direct intervention.

We attended several churches in Tulsa before joining First Methodist during the 1980 Christmas season. In December 1981, our senior pastor, Dr. L. D. Thomas, announced that the church would be refinancing the bank debt incurred to build the children's building by selling church bonds to members of the church. Even though the church had received pledges in sufficient amounts to construct the building, the fluctuating interest rates caused significant unbudgeted overruns. At the end of the service, I told Dr. Thomas that I was a securities lawyer, and I would be willing to help in the church bond offering if needed. The following day, Dr. Thomas appointed me special counsel for the church bond offering. In February 1982, the church sold $2,000,000 in church bonds to members of the church without having to pay a $60,000 outside consulting fee.

Had I not volunteered to assist First Methodist with its church bond offering, the following would not have occurred;

I would not have been appointed to be special counsel to the Church.

I would not have written the church bond offering documents.

I would not have been chair and co-chair of several First Methodist committees.

I would not have written *A Practical Guide to Church Bond Financing.*

I would not have been a member of the executive committee at First Methodist.

1994–1995: Joanne Stafford and Dub Ambrose

At a regular monthly meeting of the church executive committee in the Spring 1994, I sat next to Joanne Stafford, president of the local United Methodist Women. She was the only woman on the executive committee. After the meeting, I joked with Joanne: "Why is there a representative of United Methodist Women but not a representative of United Methodist Men? After all, equal is equal, isn't that right?" She responded, "Why don't you start a men's ministry?" That was the last thing from my mind. I was joking with her. But her comment made sense. So I went to Dr. Buskirk, our senior minister, and suggested we begin a men's ministry program. To my surprise, eleven other men in the church had approached Dr. Buskirk about the same time seeking to establish a men's ministry program. First Men was borne out of those meetings.

The twelve of us met weekly for three months trying to map out what a men's ministry program should be. We learned that one size does not fit all. Men are at different places on their faith journeys. We learned that most men today are intensely competitive, task oriented, emotionally lonely, highly individualistic, essentially friendless and spiritually hungry. We decided to host monthly meetings to hear prominent businessmen tell of how their faith informs and affects their lives in the marketplace. I love to hear the story of how Jesus helps men in their marketplace experiences. The First Men programs continue today, exploring new ways to bring the message of Christ to other men.

In late October 1995, First Men took two buses to Dallas for a Promise Keepers conference. I did not want to go, but I agreed to go when I was asked to be the "bus captain" for one of the buses. Intellectually, I was curious to see if men filled a stadium for four hours of worship on Friday evening without a game involved or women to watch. I could not believe that those same 75,000 men would show up all day Saturday to hear more sermons. And I was surprised that all 75,000 men were provided lunch in less than 30 minutes. The 1995 Dallas Promise Keepers' conference changed my life.

The conference opened with awesome praise and worship music like I had never heard. We first heard the heart wrenching testimony of James Ryle, Coach Bill McCartney's pastor, and how he served time for possession of marijuana in a prison that his father built. Dr. Tony Evans of Dallas then told how a messed up man causes a messed up family, a messed up neighborhood and a messed up nation. He observed that if we want a better nation, a better neighborhood and a better family, it all starts by becoming better men. Dr. Evans concluded by describing a scene from the movie, *Rocky IV.* When Rocky was down and almost out, his old coach Mickey, who had died, came back in a dream, urging Rocky, "Get up, get up, you bum. 'Cause Mickey loves you." But Dr. Evans said instead, "Get up, get up, you bums, 'Cause Jesus loves you." The 75,000 men stood in unison and worshipped Jesus with song and shouts of joy. I was hooked. The messages and music in Dallas spoke to me in a deep and personal way.

Without my joking comment to Joanne Stafford and her thoughtful and challenging response, the following things would not have happened:

First Men would not have come into existence.

I would not have gone to Dallas Promise Keepers in October 1995.

I would not have gone to Promise Keepers Stand in the Gap in Washington, D.C. in October 1996 where 2,000,000 men worshipped Jesus on the Main Mall.

I would not have met Coach Bill McCartney, James Ryle or Tony Evans.

I would not have written *Seeking God's Heart* or *A Treasury of Truth and Wisdom.*

As I reflect upon the past, I have come to realize that God is present in my life all the time, guiding, protecting, urging and loving me back to Him, often through His angels.

HOW AWESOME IS THAT?
TO GOD BE THE GLORY!

Cancer Confirms My Beliefs: 2012

Until recently, I had never thought about cancer, radiation, chemotherapy or stem-cell or bone marrow transfusions as applicable to me. Those things belonged to the collective experiences of others. That was before April 23, 2012, when the world as I then knew it changed. I have a new reality: I have Stage I Kappa single chain multiple myeloma. I am also an insulin dependent Type II diabetic.

The Background

For 6 months before April 23, 2012, I had not felt well. I did not have a lot of pain, just annoying issues that older people complain about. Because of my diabetes, I had frequent blood tests and full lab reports. They were normal. I experienced a number of symptoms of unknown cause, resulting in numerous X-rays and even an angiogram of my heart, all with negative results. I had a clean colonoscopy. In March, the muscles on my outer chest wall screamed with pain. This is called costochondritis. It has no known cause, but it goes away after a couple weeks. In late March, I lost strength in my left arm for no apparent reason, and I developed a case of shingles under my right arm for no apparent reason.

During this time, I had many office visits with Dr. Brent Dennis, my terrific primary care doctor. Those visits resulted in many X rays, blood tests and a variety of other tests. In early April, Dr. Dennis ordered an MRI of my chest. When the nurse closed the lid down on my chin in the MRI machine,

I totally freaked out. That MRI was stopped and rescheduled at a later date. In the mean time, Dr. Dennis referred me to Dr. Bruce Markman, an orthopedic surgeon, to examine my left arm. I scheduled an appointment for 8:30 a.m. on Good Friday, April 6.

On Wednesday, April 4, Chet Nordling, my eighty-eight-year-old uncle from Bentonville, Arkansas and my fishing buddy, called wondering if I might be able to go fishing on the White River on Friday. Initially, I told Chet that I could not, but I had promised myself earlier that if Chet ever called and wanted to go fishing, I would go if at all possible. So I called Chet back and said I would pick him up at 9:30 a.m. the following day. I cancelled my appointment with Dr. Markman on Good Friday and rescheduled it for Thursday, April 19.

Good Friday on the White River seemed to be the perfect day for fishing. As we approached the river, a huge orange moon hung low just over the hills west of the river. There was no wind, the sky was clear and there seemed no chance for rain. A heavy blanket of fog covered the water. The river was cold, crisp and friendly. It seemed to be the perfect day for catching the illusive browns.

I was wrong. The conditions were perfect for fishing but it was the worst day of catching I have ever experienced on the White River. I got two bites all day long. I did catch the 17" brown on one of those bites, but I missed the big one, which came within twenty feet of our boat as if to taunt us. By noon, Chet got tired of fishing for browns, so he fished for rainbows the rest of the day. I was stubborn and continued to fish for the big one. Even so, I do not regret canceling my orthopedic appointment with Dr. Markman scheduled for early Good Friday morning. I always have fun being on the river with Chet.

The Diagnosis

I saw Dr. Markman on Thursday, April 19. Dr. Markman ordered an X-ray of the left arm, which revealed a crack in my left elbow which I did not know was broken. Myeloma does not show up on X-rays, but Dr. Markman could see a fracture in the elbow and a dark mass around the elbow. Dr. Markman ordered an MRI of my left elbow for the following afternoon. He also ordered an open MRI of my chest for 8:00 a.m. the following Monday.

Even before the chest MRI was completed Monday morning, Dr. Dennis was preparing me to go to the hospital, because the MRI clearly showed the presence of cancer. I went straight from Dr. Dennis' office to St. Francis Hospital where I was tested for five days. Surprisingly, I was poised and completely at peace with this diagnosis and possible treatments. Normally I worry about everything.

To find out what kind of cancer I have, I was subjected to multiple tests in the hospital, including CAT scans, X-rays, MRIs, sonograms, heart echo tests, biopsies of the area around my spine where the largest lesion was located and a biopsy of the bone marrow in my hip, which proved conclusive: I have Stage I Kappa single chain multiple myeloma. This condition arises out of a disorder in my white blood cells. White blood cells produce proteins that operate our immune system. The proteins gobble up the bacteria, viruses, funguses and other impurities in our bodies we encounter each day. In multiple myeloma patients, for some unknown reason, the white blood cells get stuck open and produce too many proteins, some of which are cancerous. These extra cancerous proteins have nothing to gobble up, so they attack the patient's bones. As a result, I have holes in my bones all over my body and my immune system is compromised. Dr. Janjua, my oncologist, laughingly said that I should avoid places where sick people are, especially hospitals, salad bars and church. Fortunately, the cancer is not in any of my major organs.

Of the total myeloma population, only about 3% have the Kappa single chain type of myeloma. But because of the results from recent clinical trials, the single chain myeloma treatment has been specifically identified and quantified for most patients. Every cancer is different, and every cancer patient reacts to treatment in a different way. But if I had to have myeloma, the single chain type is the type to have, particularly after the results of these new studies.

Multiple myeloma patients do not generally present a medical or life threatening emergency, except where the cancer threatens the spinal cord. That was my case. If the spinal cord had been invaded, immediate permanent paralysis would have occurred from that point on my spine down to my feet. This condition occurs rarely, perhaps 1 of 500–600 cases annually. In my case, the largest concentration of cancer cells was between the seventh and eighth vertebra. My spinal cord had not yet been invaded, but the lesions were pressing against the spinal cord. I was a medical emergency waiting to happen any moment, but I did not know it.

The Dream Team

Dr. Dennis assembled a "Dream Team" of doctors, nurses and technicians who were exactly suited for my case: Dr. Preston Phillips, a renowned spine surgeon; Dr. Stephen Sack, a radiologist; Dr. Muhammed Janjua, an oncologist; and Dr. David Markman, a general surgeon. Each is a highly regarded expert in his field of practice, and each one is a caring, committed, highly professional doctor. Even better yet, each of these specialists can communicate complicated information in common terms. That is a special gift, especially in the highly charged emotional and uncertain atmosphere of a new cancer diagnosis. In addition, they knew that my son, Kipp, was in the last month of an internal medicine residency at Scott and White in Temple, Texas; and they welcomed Kipp into their discussions. Kipp came to Tulsa as soon as he learned of the cancer diagnosis. Kipp realized the danger of my diagnosis immediately. While Kipp was not one of my doctors, he was able to provide me with great insight into my particular situation. Kipp continues to be an invaluable resource and comfort to me.

The Treatment Plan

There are essentially three types of treatment options for myeloma: surgery, radiation and chemotherapy. Myeloma is a blood-borne systemic cancer. Myeloma attacks the entire skelital frame. There are no cancerous tumors. Myeloma leaves holes in the patient's bones all over his body. In my case, the largest concentration of lesions was located in the middle of back near my spinal cord, the most dangerous place possible.

The first treatment question was whether to do back surgery or radiation. Because the cancer was beginning to wrap itself around my spinal cord, the surgery would have been complicated and dangerous, and the recovery period would have been very long and painful. Surgery was ruled out.

The next treatment option is radiation on the specific area where the cancer was most highly concentrated: my spine, my left elbow and my left hip. Dr. Sack, my radiologist, told me that he rarely begins radiation treatments before the specific type of cancer is identified and classified. He makes an exception to that rule once in 500–600 cases. I was his 2012 exception.

I received radiation treatments each work day for 20 days, ten treatments on my entire spine, followed by ten treatments on my left hip and my left elbow done simultaneously. Radiation targets specific spots where the cancer is. The treatments took only a few minutes each.

Radiation is site specific treatment and kills cancer only in the targeted areas. Myeloma is a cancer in the blood system. Chemotherapy is the only way to kill all the cancer cells in the blood system. The chemotherapy treatment plan consists of 8 cycles of 21 days each. During the first two weeks of each three week cycle, I receive chemotherapy treatments on days 1, 4, 8 and 11. Each treatment is preceded by drawing blood to insure that I am healthy enough to take the treatment. There are no treatments during the third week of each cycle.

The treatment plan is modeled after the results of recent clinical trials, which produced results that defined the best chemical combination of drugs for the most people with exact doses involved. One-half of the chemotherapy consists of steroids, which I have been taking in a steroid pill since April 27, 2012, the first day I met Dr. Janjua. The other half is a mixture of poisons, which kill the active cancer cells as well as healthy cells too.

Based on an April 27 blood test, my number for cancerous proteins was **77.4**. The target is very simple: Drive the **77.4** down to near 0. When that occurs, doctors harvest my stem cells from my bone marrow and freeze them. A double dose of chemotherapy is administered in an effort to kill all remaining cancer cells. Then, my own stem cells are transfused back into my body and begin the building process to make my bones strong again. On July 24, 2012 the number was **2.54**. The treatments and the prayers of friends are working.

Miracles

This journey has proven to be very positive for me. I am a walking miracle, so I now have personal confirmation that God is at work continuing to create what man calls miracles. Miracles are beyond man's understanding or explanation. But God is in the miracle-making business. For God, all things are possible for those who BELIEVE.

Some who do not believe will just call me lucky. I clearly am very lucky. But the series of events leading to my diagnosis and treatment of cancer cannot be luck alone. I BELIEVE that my cancer is all about God and my response to HIS call on my life. I believe these events have been orchestrated by God, so that I can witness to world that I serve a great God. Luck has little to do with my BELIEVING that.

Here are some of the miracles I have experienced as a cancer patient:

1. I have been at peace with the diagnosis and treatment from the beginning.

2. My cancer was discovered early to permit effective treatment.

3. No back surgery was required.

4. No elbow surgery was required.

5. Thirty radiation treatments were administered one mile from my office on an outpatient basis. No out of town travel has been needed.

6. Chemotherapy treatments are being administered one mile from my office on an outpatient basis. No out of town travel has been needed.

7. The radiation and chemotherapy treatments have been given effectively and efficiently on time when promised with no unusual waiting.

8. I have been virtually pain free throughout the process.

9. I have had virtually no side effects from any of the treatments.

10. I have been able to work, even when receiving treatments.

11. I have been very busy with good paying work to do.

12. I am not paralyzed. I can walk, but I am in a back brace 24/7.

13. I have had the very best treatment, the very best doctors, nurses, technicians, and staff at the very best facilities available.

14. I feel like royalty.

15. Best of all, while my family has always been close, this experience has brought us closer than ever before.

I thank God for using my cancer for good. I am deeply grateful to friends and family. I feel warmly embraced in the loving arms of God throughout this journey. My family has been unbelievable, especially Claudia, who has had to shoulder the burden of being my cook and driver and everything else, in addition to all her other chores. How can I ever thank her enough? I will be forever grateful for this experience, which could have been horrible but which turned into a journey of wonder, mystery and awe for the God of creation.

Conclusion

God is in control. He loves me and wants the very best for me. I have placed my trust, hope and joy in Him. I trust Him completely. I am filled with His peace and His joy.

This I Believe!

Part V:

THE RIVER

The River

I have often wondered why fishing for trout in the clear cold waters of the White River in Arkansas has so captured my excitement, why the long cast of my sculpin into the deep dark pool along the rocky shore holds my fascination. I have also wondered why the river draws me back, keeps me interested and captures my thoughts, desires, hopes and dreams from the very core of my being. It is not the fishing that draws me, but the river itself that calms me and makes me feel close to God.

The allure of the river is magical, mysterious, even metaphysical. There is something very calming, spiritual, even holy about the river. The river is constantly in motion, sometimes calm, wide and slow; sometimes raging, narrow and fast; sometimes shallow and swift, sometimes deep and mercurial. The river bends and shifts, turns and tumbles, glides and rages. The river is like life itself. Just when you believe you have it under control, storm clouds gather, thunder rumbles, lightning strikes, the sky bursts open and I am thrown into uncertainty.

My first time on the White River was in 1987 when my three new law partners and I took our five sons fishing. It was the last weekend of September. When we got on the river that Saturday morning, the temperature hovered around freezing. Kipp, my 11 year old son, wore five layers of clothes when the day began, but by the end of the day, he was wearing only a T-shirt. His first cast was rewarded with a nice rainbow, and we were both hooked. There is something magical about fishing with Kipp.

Since then, I have returned to the river at least once a year. I took my daughter, Laura, to the river during the summer after her second year of law school. Our guide was a huge red neck wearing overalls with an intimating full red beard. He tried to get under Laura's skin, but she was too tough for him. The guide required Laura to fish with live crickets and bait her own hook, which I have never seen since. Before the day was over, she too was hooked on the river. Laura caught more than seventy rainbows that day.

I later took my wife, Claudia, fishing on the river. She got bored after catching almost a hundred rainbows. I have never been bored catching fish. I have introduced many people to the adventure of fishing on the White River, and all of them have been back for more. It is fun on the river, but it is much more than fun to me. It is magical, mystical, mysterious, even sacred to be on the river.

Four years ago, I had the great pleasure of introducing my four-year-old grandson, Eli, to the river. I thought that Eli was a couple years too young, but I was wrong. We prepared for our trip by getting Eli his own Spiderman vest and matching fishing pole. I taught Eli to cast in our front yard in Tulsa. When we arrived at Stetson's, we were greeted by Jerry Killabrew, our handsome bare-foot guide. Jerry knows the river, knows fishing and is very good with young boys. When releasing the fish back into the river, Jerry never takes the hook out, saying that the fish will have a better chance of surviving with the hook in its mouth. Eli caught at least sixty rainbow that first day. The following day, Eli and I were guided by Josh, Jerry's friend. Jerry told Eli to tell Josh he fishes like a girl. Eli did. Josh turned red, then rolled over laughing. Eli and I have a great time fishing together. On our trip back to Tulsa, Eli asked if he could invite twenty of his best friends from Georgia to attend his fifth birthday party on the river.

Eli and I go to the White River at least once annually now. Each year, Eli catches more fish than I do. Last year he caught a 6 lb. 2 oz. brown. It was the biggest brown I have seen caught. He now tells his friends: "Fred goes fishing, but I go catching." I cannot wait to take his little brother, Max, now age three, to the river next year. Fishing produces magical memories.

I fish out of Cotter Trout Dock, owned by Ron and Debbie Gamble, where I first met the river. The one day float trip from Cotter gives the fisherman the most variety on the river, the longest float (14 miles) and the most diverse scenery and diversity of fishing experiences. The trip begins at 7:00 a.m. and ends at 4:00 p.m. We always see eagles, blue herring, deer and other wildlife. Every day on the river is a great day.

I am haunted by the river. I am captured by the moment, knowing that the ancient call to purpose is to fish for the hearts and souls of others who do not yet know Jesus, who do not yet believe, who have not yet surrendered to the Son of the God of Creation, the God of the River. We are called to be fishers of men!

Yet we do not surrender or bow down to worship Him until a crisis beyond our understanding and control rocks our very core and draws us back to the God of grace, back to the heart of God, back to the hope, power, joy and peace of God. That is when the River of Life becomes real, when we choose to surrender and worship Him, when we hear the call and feel the tug of God's nudge for us to believe.

I feel the river calling me to full surrender, but for some reason, I want to live life on my own terms through my own efforts. What keeps me from full surrender? Why do I resist, reject, even ignore Him? I choose my way, not His. Why do I not fall down and worship Him?

I think doubts and pride are hard wired into mankind's DNA, that we want to do life on our own terms as we want it, not as God would choose it for us. Inevitably, we do seek Him when we come to the end of ourselves and find that God has been waiting for us there all along. Ultimately, we cannot do this thing called life without including Him in it. It simply does not work. But we try anyway.

Still I am drawn to the river, if not to the God of the River of Life. I am captivated by the glory of nature, if not the wonder of nature's Author. I am in awe of waters, gently, inexplicably, inevitably flowing on a journey, moving through God's Holy Valley to His Holy Presence. I seek streams of living water and fountains of cleansing, refreshing, healing waters. But most of all, I seek Him. I hear His call: "Draw near." "Follow Me." "Come to Me." "Rest in My arms." "Choose My peace." "Choose My joy." "Choose Me." **"Believe."**

God's ancient people were haunted by the River too. The Tigris and the Euphrates bordered the Fertile Crescent, from which man's beginnings can be traced. Moses was plucked out of a basket in the Nile, later to lead God's people out of slavery and into freedom to the land of milk and honey. Jesus received the affirmation of His Father while standing waist deep in waters at Bethsada. There He received the Holy Spirit and began a three-year ministry that led to the cross, to His death and resurrection and to our hope for life eternal with

Him. After receiving God's blessing, Jesus picked fishermen as His first disciples, not high priests or holy men, but ordinary men who knew the power of the river and the wonder, awe and majesty of God's creation.

The river was present in the Garden of Eden before the Fall of Man.

"In the middle of the garden were the tree of life and the tree of the knowledge of good and evil. A river watering the garden flowed from Eden: from there it was separated into four headwaters." Genesis 2:9–10

The Jordan River was used by God to affirm God's blessings upon Joshua.

"And the Lord said to Joshua, 'Today I will begin to exalt you in the eyes of all Israel, so they may know that I am with you as I was with Moses.' Tell the priests who carry the arc of the covenant: 'When you reach the edge of the Jordan's waters, go and stand in the river.'" Joshua 3:7–8 **"So Joshua commanded the priests, 'Come out of the Jordan.' And the priests came out of the river carrying the arc of the covenant of the Lord."** Joshua 4:17–18

The river is always present when Scripture refers to the city of God.

"There is a river whose streams make glad the city of God, the holy place where the Most High dwells." Psalm 46:4

A river played a central role in the life of a Presbyterian minister and his family in the short autobiographical story,

A River Runs Through It. The story takes place in the Big Sky Country of Montana. There are two boys in the family. Norman, the older boy and the author of the story, is serious, intelligent and a lover of literature, like his father. Norman is like the good son in the story of the Prodigal. Norman receives the inheritance, his father's love of literature, but unlike the Biblical Prodigal, Norman leaves home to teach at the University of Chicago. Paul, the younger boy, is handsome, rebellious, fun loving and likes to gamble, drink and party with the ladies. Paul never leaves the physical proximity of his father's home, but Paul clearly lives in the far country, never far from his father's love. Paul becomes a journalist for the local paper and continues to party. His fun loving ways contributed to his being murdered at a young age.

The boys and their father have one thing in common: trout fishing on the Big Barefoot River. Norman recalls his last fishing trip with his father and brother like this:

"We sat on the bank as the river went by. As always, it was making sounds to itself, and now it made sounds to us. It would be hard to find three men sitting side-by-side who knew better what a river was saying.

"On the Big Barefoot River above the mouth of Belmont Creek, the banks are fringed by large Ponderosa pines. In the slanting sun of late afternoon, the shadows of great branches reach from across the river, and the trees took the river in their arms. The shadows continued up the bank, until they included us.

"A river, though, has so many things to say that it is hard to know what it says to each of us. As we were packing our tackle and fish in the car, Paul repeated, "Just give me three more years." At the time, I was surprised at the repetition, but later I realized that the river somewhere, sometime, must have told me, too, that he would receive no such gift. ... [Paul was murdered soon after this trip.]

Later, Norman and his father were remembering Paul:

"I've said I've told you all I know. If you push me far enough, all I really know is that [Paul] was a fine fisherman."

"You know more than that," my father said. "He was beautiful."

"Yes," I said, "he was beautiful. He should have been—you taught him..."

The story ends when Norman returns to Montana after retiring as a Professor of Literature at the University of Chicago. All his family have passed, but Montana is where Norman grew up, and that is where he calls "home." It is natural for a man to come home to the place of his youth at the end of his life, to the memories of family and friends, wiser, weathered, even worn down, but still hopeful.

Norman ends by saying:

"It is those we live with and love and should know that elude us...."

"Eventually, all things merge into one, and a river runs through it."

"The river was cut by the world's great flood and runs over rocks from the basement of time. On some of the rocks are timeless raindrops. Under the rocks are the words, and some of the words are theirs.

"I am haunted by waters." See *A River Runs Through It and Other Stories,* pp. 101–104.

I, too, am haunted by the river and by its waters, full of life and ever-changing, though constant and changeless as anything God ever created. The river connects us, separates us, feeds us and floods us. The river flows, and we flow with it, whether carried by our own will or moved by the timeless flow of time itself. The river is essential to our lives, and often takes away our sense of security, sometimes even our very own lives. We cannot live life without it, but we cannot tame or control it either.

The river is a symbol of the cycle of life itself. Sometimes, the river roars down a steep mountain gorge with the fury of a spring thunderstorm, destroying everything it its path. At other times, the river meanders gently through the deep holes where the big browns feed. But always and forever, the river is in constant motion, continuing to create and sustain all forms of life. The river is a symbol of hope, restoration, regeneration, recreation and renewal.

As the shadows fall on the life of the fisherman, standing alone waist deep in the crystal cold waters of the river, man comes to know that surrender is the only way to real freedom, the only way to be in His presence. Ultimately, man's search for purpose leads to belief, and belief leads to surrender, but only after man concludes that he is not God, and he cannot achieve joy or peace without including God in his life. Ultimately, man finds meaning and purpose from the abundance that comes from the throne of God delivered by the river of God's incomprehensible grace.

The river watered the Garden of Eden and separated the tree of life from the tree of the knowledge of good and evil. The river is always present in the city of God. The river flows from the throne of God.

"Then the angel showed me the river of the water of life, as clear as crystal, flowing from the throne of God and of the Lamb down the middle of the great street of the city. On each side of the river stood the tree of life, bearing twelve crops of fruit, yielding its fruit every month. And the leaves of the tree are for the healing of the nations. No longer will there be any curse. The throne of God and of the Lamb will be in the city, and his servants will serve him. They will see his face, and his name will be on their foreheads. There will be no night. They will not need a lamp or the light of the sun, for the Lord God will give them light. And they will reign for ever and ever." Revelation 22:1–5

Finally, the river symbolizes what I believe: There is a God who created all, who is all knowing, all powerful and always available. My God is active, alive, real and personal. He loves me personally, even when I leave Him out of my life. He wants me to spend time with Him in His presence. He is the source for every good and perfect gift. All of God's blessings come from His throne. The river is the means by which God showers us with His joy, peace, grace, abundance and hope. If I intentionally and constantly choose Him, I will receive His blessings beyond belief. In the end, all things do merge into God, and the river of His blessings will flow freely from His throne with no end.

THIS I BELIEVE!

About the Author

Frederick K. Slicker is a business lawyer in Tulsa, Oklahoma. He holds a Bachelor of Arts (BA) in mathematics from the University of Kansas (1965), a Juris Doctor (JD) with highest distinction from the University of Kansas School of Law (1968) and a Master of Laws (LL.M) from Harvard Law School (1973). He has practiced law since 1968, primarily in the areas of securities compliance, mergers and acquisitions, franchise compliance, purchase and sale of businesses, general business organizations and general business transactions. He serves as an independent mediator for business issues. He is a frequent speaker at continuing legal education programs on subjects in his areas of practice and on legal ethics and professionalism topics.

Fred has been recognized by his peers as a Best Lawyer in America in the areas of mergers and acquisitions and franchise law, and he has been an AV peer-selected lawyer by Martindale-Hubble for more than ten years. He was the recipient of the prestigious 2010 Neil Bogan Award for Professionalism and the Tulsa County Bar President's Award in 2005, 2007, 2009 and 2010–2011 for his work on professionalism and grievance matters. Fred is an active men's ministry leader at First United Methodist Church in Tulsa.

In addition to *This I Believe*, Fred has written the following books: *A Practical Guide to Church Bond Financing*, a guide for churches to conduct church bond programs in compliance with federal and state securities laws; *Angels All Around*, a memoir of his early life and in the practice of law; *Seeking God's Heart, A Devotional Journey through the Psalms;* and *A Treasury of Truth and Wisdom*, a collection of Biblically-based aphorisms intended to inspire, motivate and encourage the reader to lead a life beyond success to significance.

Please feel free to contact Fred at Slicker Law Firm, P.C., 4444 East 66th Street, Suite 201, Tulsa, OK 74136-4206; phone: 918-496-9020; fax: 918-496-9024; email: fred@slickerlawfirm.com; and website: www.slickerlawfirm.com.